EAT UP AND CLEAN UP IN A TRADITIONAL WAY

KSHAMA RAO

I dedicate this book to god, my ancestors, and the readers of this book.

Contents

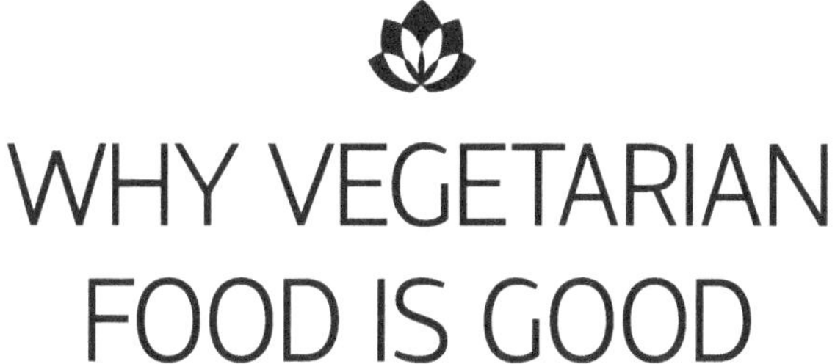

CHAPTER ONE

WHY VEGETARIAN FOOD IS GOOD

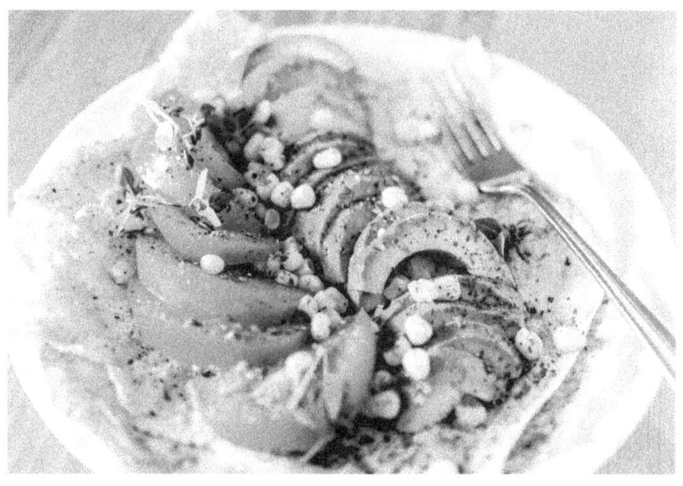

In Bhagavad Gita, it is mentioned that vegetarian food is 'Satvik'. Humans don't need non-vegetarian food and we have a choice of vegetarian food. Our body is not designed for a non-vegetarian diet. Vegetarian food is full of nutrients and supports spiritual growth. Even Buddhism and Jainism support this theory. A vegetarian diet is a violence-free diet and it really provides all the necessary complete nutrition including proteins. According to studies plant-based diets are linked with lower levels of cholesterol, obesity, and blood pressure. You can slowly start weaning off from non-vegetarian food if you are a non-vegetarian by having a cheat meal once in a while. I am not forcing anyone to be a vegetarian, it is completely their choice but this is just my view.

CHAPTER TWO

DIET PLAN FOR A GIRL WHO HAS HIT PUBERTY

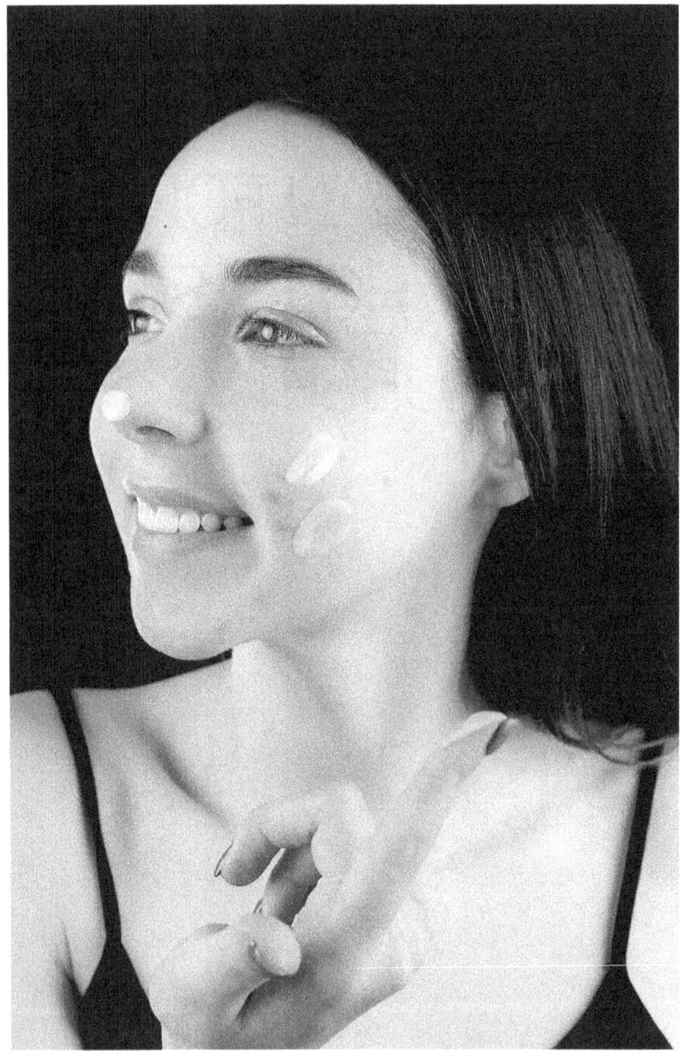

A girl, who has hit puberty should consume more iron, calcium, and protein as she has started menstruating. She should avoid consuming unhealthy fats. Here is her diet plan.

EARLY MORNING

A glass of lukewarm water

BREAKFAST

Vermicelli upma/Multigrain sandwich/Chapathi and sabzi and a glass of milk

LUNCH

Dal fry and rice/raw salad/sabzi/ with a bowl of curd with chia seeds or flax seeds or pulao and raita

EVENING

Bhelpuri

DINNER

Vegetable soup/salad/Dal and rice/Multigrain Chapathi and sabzi

Avoid restaurant food, biscuits, maida, whole milk, cream, carbonated drinks, refined oil, bakery food, processed food, and noodles. Don't eat too much spicy food. Don't skip your breakfast.

Consume more seasonal fruits and vegetables, pulses, mustard oil, and low-fat milk. Be physically active.

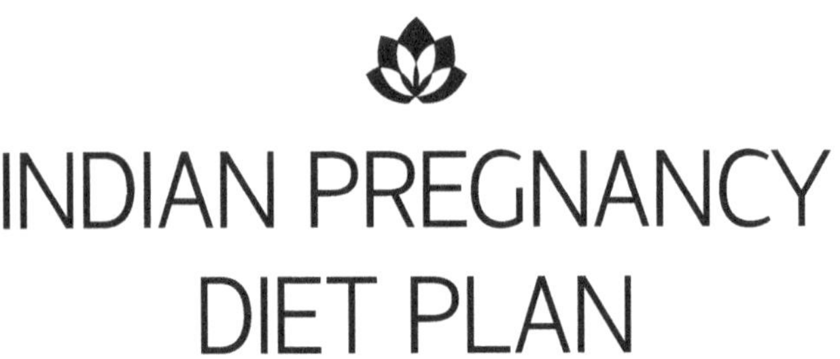

INDIAN PREGNANCY DIET PLAN

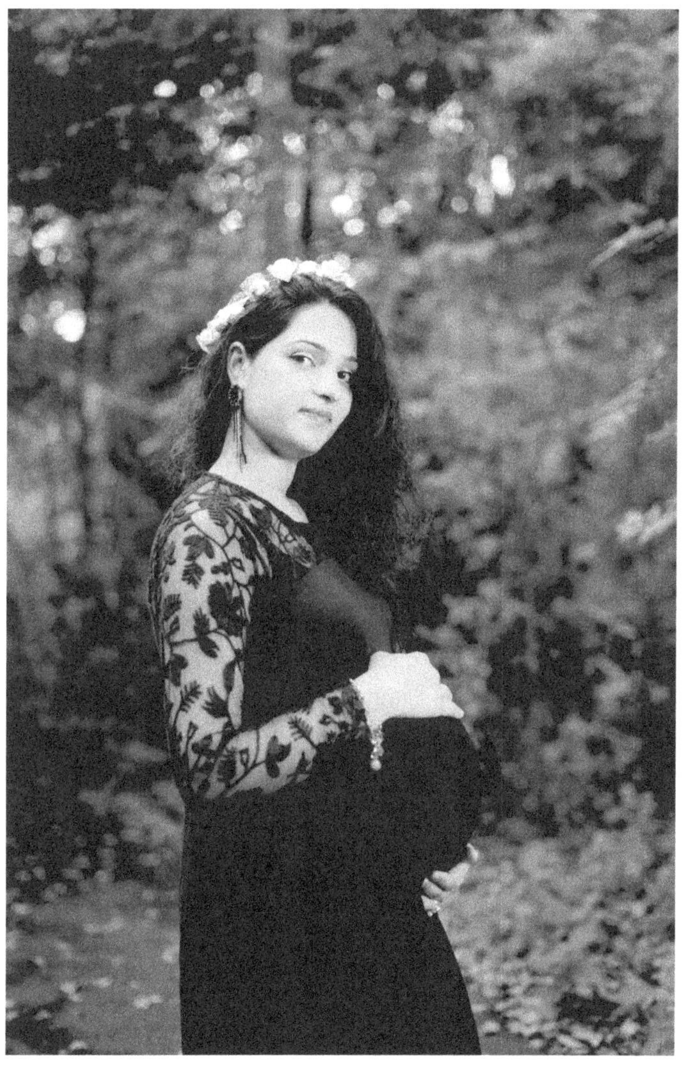

You should consume a balanced diet when you are pregnant. It is important to keep your body hydrated. You should include liquids in your diet. This diet plan provides all the nutrients required for the mother and the baby in her womb.

PRE-BREAKFAST SNACK

Milkshake

BREAKFAST

A bowl of mixed fruits/Whole wheat toast with butter/ paratha/vegetable cutlet/cheese toast/Rice vermicelli

MID-MORNING SNACK

Tomato soup/Carrot and beetroot soup/creamy spinach soup

LUNCH

Roti sabzi and dal and a bowl of curd/vegetable or paneer paratha with raita/Rice and sambar and curd rice

EVENING SNACK

Vermicelli with vegetables/vegetable samosa/green tea

DINNER

Roti with dal, sabzi and a glass of buttermilk/Paratha

You should consume Folic acid supplements. Make sure you consume lots of dry fruits. You should avoid consuming raw papaya, colocasia, Tulsi, Aloe Vera, and Pineapple. These are not safe to consume during pregnancy. Visit your doctor every month and taking her consultation is very important.

CHAPTER FOUR

INDIAN VEGETARIAN DIET PLAN FOR LACTATING WOMAN

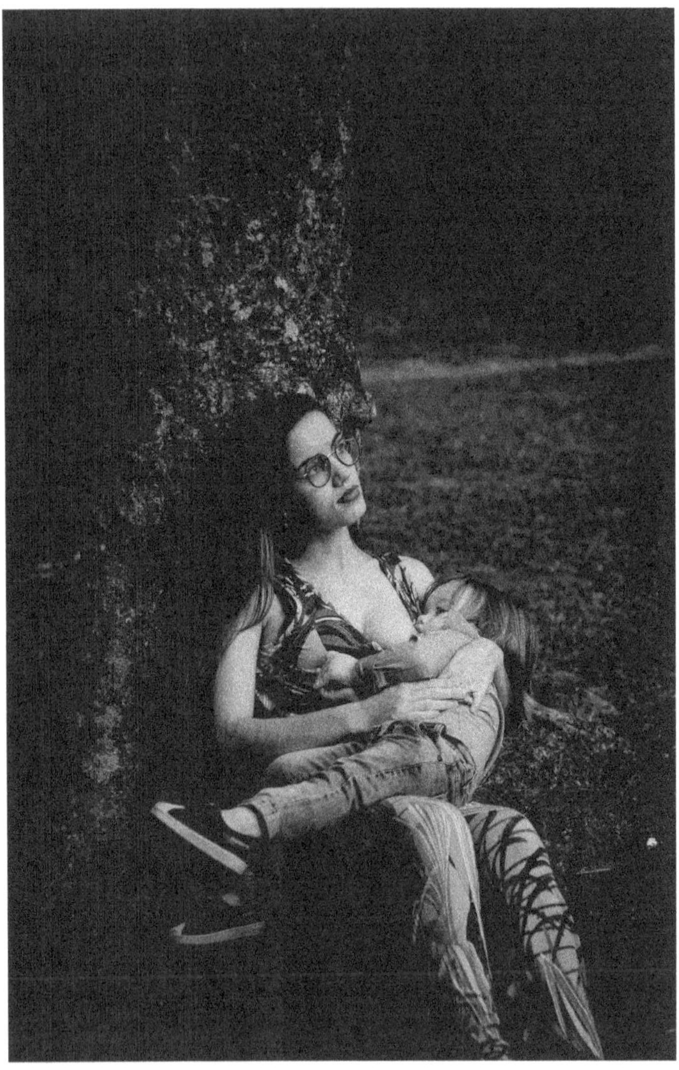

The quality of your breast milk depends on the food you consume. Your newborn baby derives complete nutrition from your breast milk. Breast milk promotes the brain development of your baby. It increases the immunity of your baby. Breastfeeding is beneficial for the mother too as it helps her uterus regain its normal size and calms her hormones. Here is a sample diet plan.

BREAKFAST

Poha/Upma/Paratha/Cheese sandwich and a big glass of Elaichi milk or kheer and gondh laddus or Panjiri

MID-MORNING

Orange juice/apple juice/pomegranate juice/Ragi porridge/coconut water/herbal tea and fruit salad with chia seeds or flax seeds

LUNCH

Chapatis with vegetable and paneer sabzi/Rice and vegetable with sprouts sambar and dal fry, raita

EVENING

A big glass of milk/cracker biscuit/Wheat or ragi biscuits/ digestive biscuits

DINNER

Vegetable soup with Lunch recipes repeated

BEFORE GOING TO BED

A big glass of milk

You should drink lots of water.

TIPS

It is important to walk for at least half an hour. You should even burp your baby. Try to sleep for eight hours per day. Happy parenting!

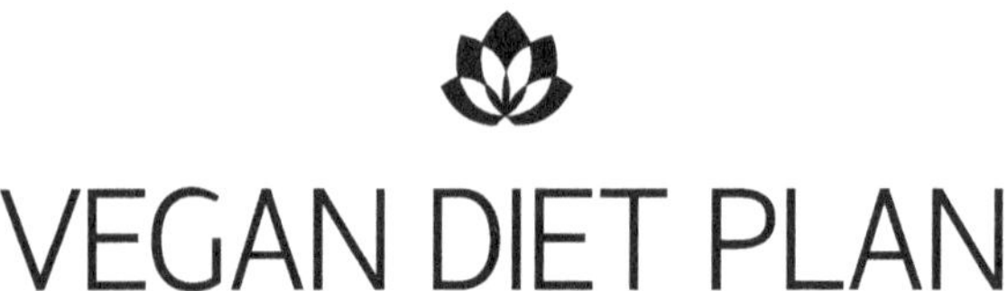

CHAPTER FIVE

VEGAN DIET PLAN

The vegan diet has many health benefits. It is a diet plan where we quit eating all animal products. It helps in lowering BMI and LDL Cholesterol. Here is a sample of the diet plan.

BREAKFAST

Sauteed mushrooms/sweet potatoes/fruits/whole-grain toast

LUNCH

Salad and whole-grain pasta/vegetable and black bean burger/black beans and vegetables fry with rice

SNACKS

Air-popped popcorn/fruit salad

DINNER

Chickpea tacos

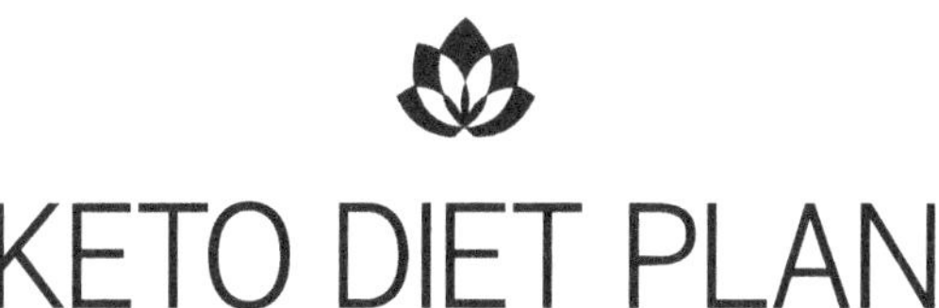

KETO DIET PLAN

The Keto diet allows you to consume fatty items. Ketosis is a state where your body uses fat as energy instead of carbs. It lowers the levels of the hormone insulin. The process of weight loss begins in three days and it may take a little longer if you are too obese. Here is a sample diet plan of the Indian keto diet.

PRE-BREAKFAST

A glass of Lauki juice/Lemon with honey juice/wheatgrass juice/ajwain water/carrot juice

BREAKFAST

Paneer paratha/Rawa idli with coconut chutney/cheese pakora

LUNCH

Paneer and mixed vegetables except potato with zero oil/ paneer paratha

SNACK

Green tea and dry fruits

DINNER

Soup/Salad/fruit/paneer stuffed capsicum

CHAPTER SEVEN

MEDITARRENEAN DIET PLAN

The Mediterranean diet plan is good for our heart and liver health. It is full of vegetables, fruits, and salads. Here is a diet plan.

PRE-BREAKFAST

Lemon water warm/Warm water with honey/

BREAKFAST

1 bowl of oatmeal/Muesli/Fruit salad

MID-MORNING

1 Fruit/salad/Vegetable soup

LUNCH

Vegetable wrap/Bean salad/Whole grain bread and vegetables sandwich/Zucchini boats with vegetables/Chapati and peas curry/Whole wheat pizza

SNACK

Salad/Whole grain pasta with vegetables/Mushroom soup/Paneer and vegetable salad

DINNER

Stir-fried vegetables/Sweet potatoes/Chapati with lentils or Chole/Vegetable kababs

BEDTIME

Yogurt with Chia or Flax seeds/Nuts/Raisins

CHAPTER EIGHT

INDIAN VEGETARIAN DIET PLAN TO REDUCE PCOS

Weight loss can be challenging for women with PCOS (Polycystic ovarian syndrome). This condition may cause excess hair growth, acne, and weight gain. You should eat a fiber-rich and antioxidant-rich diet. Irregular periods, male pattern baldness, excess hair gain on the skin, weight gain, headaches, and dark patches on the skin are symptoms that you might be having PCOS. This condition may increase your chance of getting chronic diseases like Fatty liver, High blood pressure, or even endometrial cancer. You should eat more vegetables and avoid fatty foods. Here is a diet plan.

EARLY MORNING

Green tea/Herbal tea/Lemon tea/

BREAKFAST

Ragi or Rawa Dosa with coconut chutney with a glass of orange juice/ Brown rice Idly with coconut and mint/ Upma chutney

MID_MORNING SNACK

1 Fruit/vegetable soup

LUNCH

Brown rice and Rassam with vegetable stir fry and curd/ Brown rice pulao and raita/Brown rice and sambar with sprouts and vegetables in it and curd/Multigrain chapati, dal and sabzi with curd/Methi thepla with curd and vegetable curry

SNACK

Fruits/Whole wheat bread toast/Baked cutlets or tikkis with green tea/Multigrain biscuits

PRE-DINNER

Tomato soup/Carrot soup

DINNER

Wheat Dosa/Chapati and vegetable Kurma/Chapati and Chana masala with salad/Chapati and paneer curry/Moong and peas khichdi

INDIAN VEGETARIAN DIET PLAN FOR TYPE -1 DIABETICS

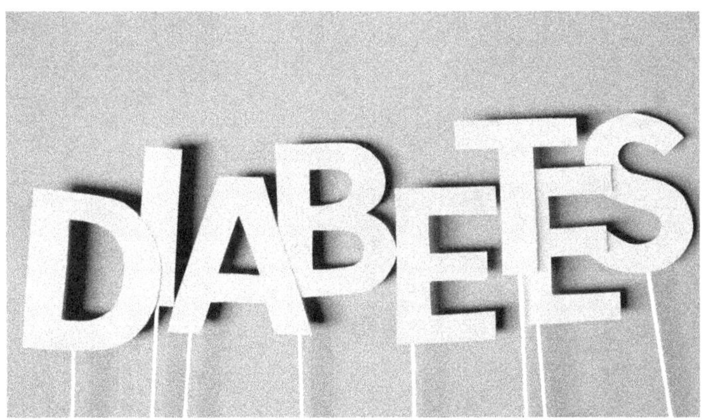

People suffering from diabetes have a double risk of getting a heart attack. extreme thirst and hunger, bruises that heal slowly, and itchy skin are symptoms of diabetes. Diabetes doesn't mean that you should give up eating your

favorite foods like rice or sweets. Here is a sample diet plan.
PRE-BREAKFAST
Sugarless tea with Marie biscuits
BREAKFAST
Methi or Palak paratha/Roti with Paneer sabzi/Vegetable Upma/Poha
MID-MORNING
Any fruit other than mango and banana
LUNCH
One roti without ghee with dal and sabzi, salad
EVENING SNACK
Bhel puri
DINNER
Salad, 2 rotis with lauki sabzi
You can drink one cup of warm elaichi milk before going to bed.

CHAPTER TEN

INDIAN DIET PLAN FOR TYPE TWO DIABETES

You should consume foods that release energy slowly. You should avoid eating junk food and skipping breakfast. Deep sleep, stress management, exercise, and dietary habits can help reverse Type two diabetes. Here is a sample diet plan.

PRE-BREAKFAST

Methi detox water

BREAKFAST

Vegetable paratha/one to two whole-wheat toast sandwiches with a cup of low-fat tea or coffee/Idly chutney/Poha/Upma/Vegetable cutlet with tea or coffee

MID-MORNING

Low glycemic fruits

LUNCH

1 or 2 Chapatis or multigrain rotis with sabzi, dal, and curd/Dal paratha with curd/Paneer paratha without oil and salad/Wheat pasta with vegetables and a plate of salad

EVENING SNACKS

Fruits and curd/Ragi khakhra/Behl Puri
DINNER
1 to 2 Chapatis with vegetables and salads with a bowl of
dal and curd/Besan Cheela with a bowl of dal and salad
or sprouts/Salad and Ragda Pattice/Multigrain Rotis with
Karela sabzi and salad

CHAPTER ELEVEN

INDIAN VEGETARIAN DIET PLAN FOR BLOOD PRESSURE

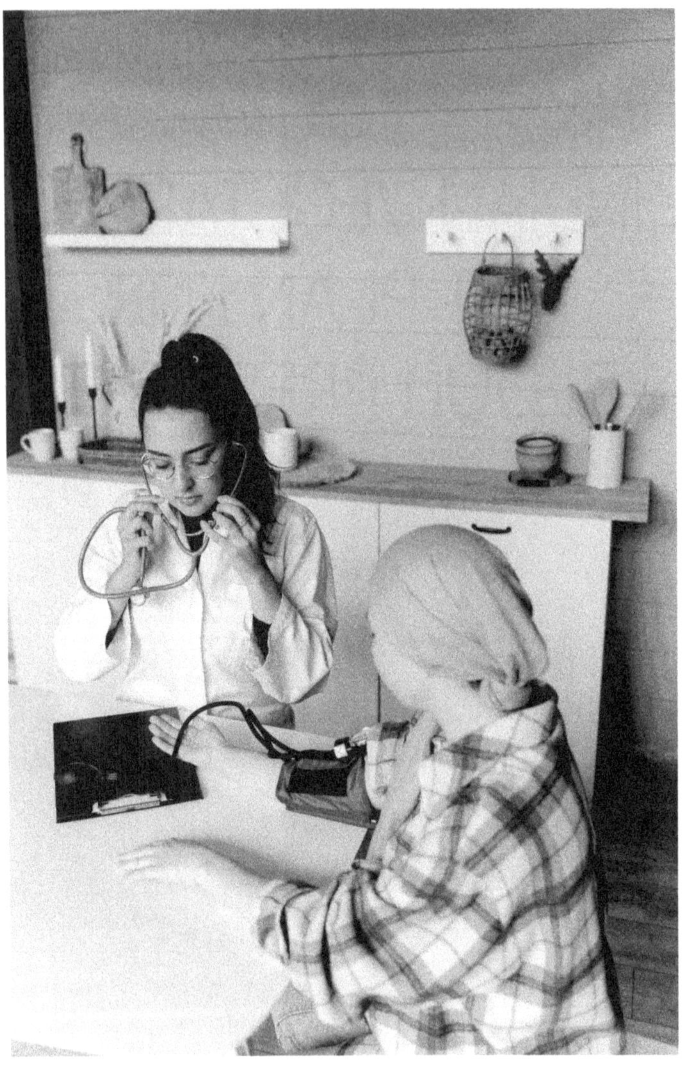

Blood pressure is a lifestyle-borne condition. It is a silent killer. It causes damage to the wall of our arteries.

Here is a sample diet plan from which you can control BP.
BREAKFAST
One handful of roasted Flax seed/Carrot or Spinach Paratha
MID-MORNING
Fruit salad (Banana, Orange, Watermelon, and Guava)
LUNCH
Brown rice pulao and raita/Whole grain roti, sabzi, and dal with a plate of salad
EVENING
Green tea with Bel puri
DINNER
Wheat flour roti with dal

CHAPTER TWELVE

INDIAN VEGETARIAN DIET PLAN FOR GERD

Nutrition is important to manage GERD. Consuming frequent small meals will be helpful. GERD is also known as Gastroesophageal reflux disease. Here is a sample diet plan that helps you cope with GERD.

PRE-BREAKFAST

Aloe Vera juice

BREAKFAST

Upma/Poha/Vegetable vermicelli Upma/Chapati with sabzi and roti

MID-MORNING

Fruit salad/Coconut water/Gree tea/Herbal tea

LUNCH

Chapati, sabzi, and dal with curd

SNACK

Green tea with Bhel puri or Vegetable soup

DINNER

Chapati, sabzi, dal and curd

TIPS

Do not sleep immediately after having meals.

Manage stress by yoga.

Try to manage a healthy weight.

Avoid spicy food.
Minimize outside eating.
Do not wear skin-tight clothes.

• 25 •

INDIAN VEGETARIAN DIET PLAN FOR POT BELLY

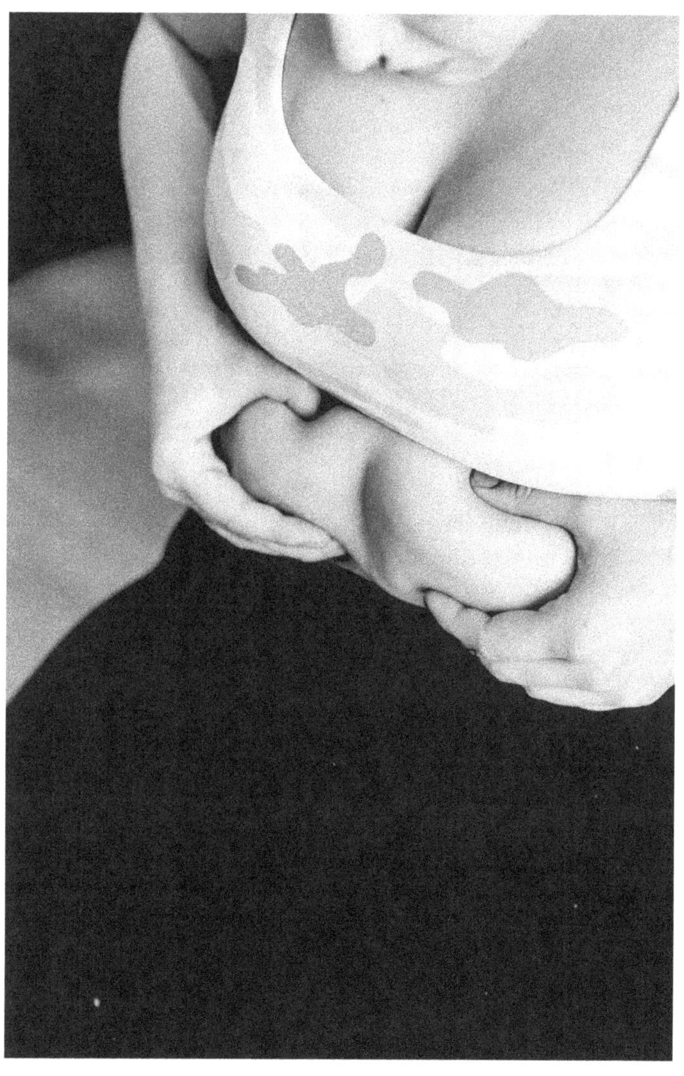

Is your belly size not reducing? Liver problems, hypothyroidism, unhealthy diet and lifestyle, stress, and poor sleep quality may cause pot belly. Eating healthy is a good start. We should eat less carbohydrates and more healthy fats. So, do you want a flat belly? Here is a diet plan for you.

EARLY MORNING

Nuts of your choice

BREAKFAST

Brown bread sandwich with a glass of orange juice and a banana

MID-MORNING

Salad/fruit of your choice/two to three whole wheat crackers

LUNCH

Brown rice with vegetable curry and salad/a bowl of poha with one roti and dal, salad/ Chickpea and vegetable salad/ Khichdi with raita or curd/Rajma rice with Raita

SNACKS

Green tea and sprouts or Khakhra/Paneer tikka

DINNER

One roti with sabzi, salad, and lentil soup

You can have a glass of milk before going to bed.

TIPS

Drink lots of water.

Avoid carbohydrates and consume more protein and fiber.

Avoid consuming sugar.

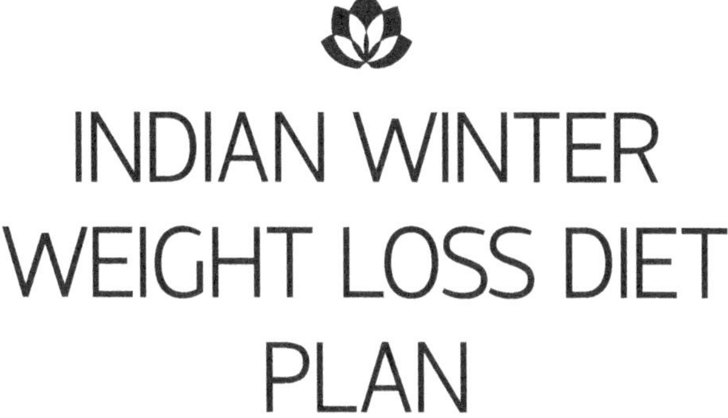

INDIAN WINTER WEIGHT LOSS DIET PLAN

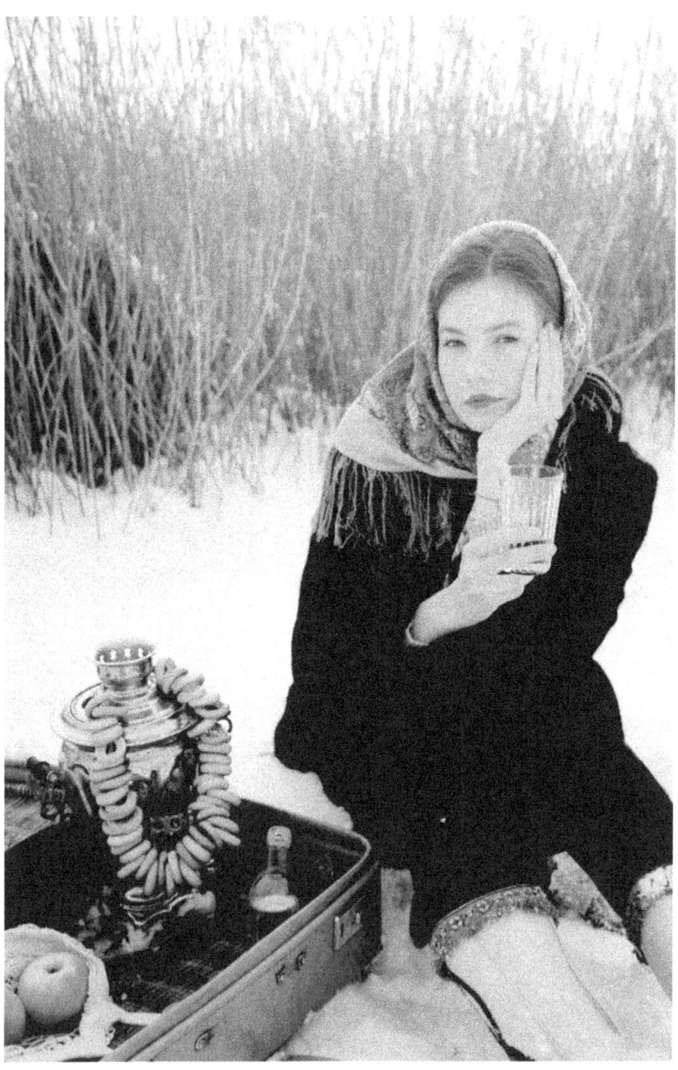

Do you want to lose weight during the winters? Here is
a sample diet plan.

EARLY MORNING
Warm Lemon water with ginger slices
BREAKFAST
A bowl of fruits with curd/A bowl of cereals with a glass of milk
LUNCH
A bowl of brown rice with vegetable stir fry, a bowl of salad with one roti, and a small Katorii of daal
SNACK
Green tea with multigrain biscuits
DINNER
Two rotis with a bowl of daal, paneer, and mixed vegetable sabzi
You should consume plenty of seasonal fruits in the winters.

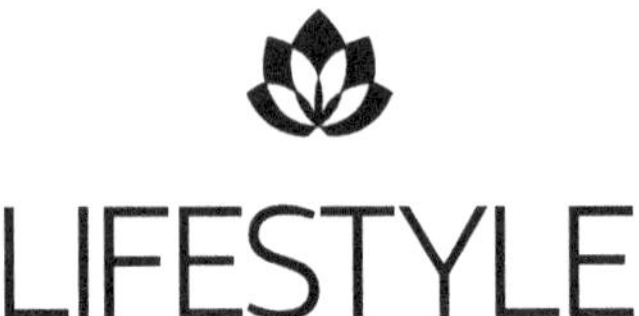

LIFESTYLE

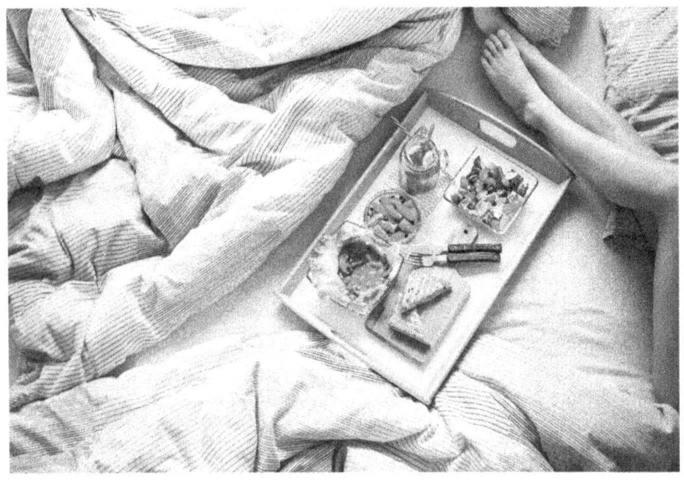

Our body is our temple. We should take care of it. We should not abuse our bodies. A good lifestyle will lengthen our lifespan. Here are a few tips.

DRINK MORE WATER

We should drink three liters of water a day. Drinking more water fills our stomachs.

GET ENOUGH SLEEP

Lack of sleep causes premature aging.

EXERCISE

Exercising increases our life span. Choose climbing stairs instead of taking the elevator. Work out daily and pick a sport of your liking.

EAT FRUITS AND VEGETABLES

Include a variety of fruits and vegetables in your diet. Choose from different colors.

HAVE HOBBIES

Travel often. Find your passion and make it your career. Fix your work time and spare time for your hobbies. Get mentors and set role models. A self-care routine is a must. Periodically visit a therapist and speak out.

REMOVE NEGATIVE PEOPLE FROM YOUR LIFE

Remove overly negative or critical people from your life. Remove people who don't respect you from your life. Spend more time with like-minded people.

MEDITATE

Take deep breaths. This will expand your abdomen. Most of us are not breathing properly.

FALL IN LOVE

Find your soulmate.

DO KIND DEEDS

Help the needy people.

BE GRATEFUL

Express gratitude for everything you have in life. Keep upgrading yourself.

QUIT COMPLAINING

Stop complaining and start working on your problem. Let the past go. Try to forgive people who did wrong to you. Make new friends.

BE EMPATHETIC AND COMPASSIONATE

Show compassion to people and don't bad mouth them.

Connect with your old friends.

DECLUTTER

Throw unwanted things and clean your house.

• 34 •